What Should I Eat?

The Secrets to Healthy Food That No One is Talking About and a Scientific Approach to a Healthy Diet

Table of Contents

Disclaimer

This book is not intended as a substitute for the medical advice of physicians. The reader should regularly consult a physician in matters relating to his/her health and particularly with respect to any symptoms that may require diagnosis or medical attention. Please note that the information contained herein is for educational and entertainment purposes only. Every attempt has been made to provide accurate, current, and complete information. No warranty of any kind is expressed or implied. Readers acknowledge that the author is not engaging in the

I want to thank you and congratulate you for downloading the book, "What should I eat? The Secrets to Healthy Food That No One is Talking About and a Scientific Approach to a Healthy Diet".

This book contains proven steps and strategies on how to successfully choose healthy food from a well researched standpoint. Almost anyone can benefit greatly from this diet and now it's your turn. Follow this guide and you are sure to start looking and feeling better in no time!

Thanks again for downloading this book and I hope you enjoy it!

Introduction

The question of what we should eat is not surprising, considering that the media inundates us with advertisements on food products that claim to be clean and healthy. What makes things is worse is that some people who claim to be experts have different perspectives on nutrition than what we hear through the media. Most often, these perspectives are inconsistent and conflicting.

For example, one of the biggest lies we've been told is about fat. For a long time, we have been instilled with the idea through people close to us, from the media, and health and nutrition experts that fat is bad for our health and that we should eat low-fat foods. They told us that too much fat would lead to an increase in cholesterol levels and to negative health consequences, including an increase in body fat. We believed, and we stayed away from fatty foods. Avoiding all fatty foods, however, did not stop people from gaining weight.

So, we continued the search for the culprit. In avoiding fatty foods, we turned to carbohydrates, which nutritionists now say are unhealthy. Certain types of carbohydrates are indeed unhealthy due to their compositions. Sugar and starch are examples of this. These carbohydrates are high in calories and have a big effect on blood sugar.

Now, calories are not bad in themselves. Calories are simply energy for our bodies. However, carbohydrates are an energy source that is harmful when taken in excessive amounts because the body stores them as fat. As a result, people who consume too many carbs are overweight and suffer from diabetes and a myriad of other illnesses. We find food products rich in carbohydrates in abundance in the center aisles of supermarkets and groceries. They are everywhere! Then we learned that not all carbs are "bad carbs".

The search for a food to blame did not stop with carbohydrates. We became attached to high protein food and low carbohydrate diet, which again, was not all it was cracked up to be.

The fact is, we have a propensity to get attached to one nutrient in our diet and exclude everything else, for focus on excluding one so much that we ignore everything else. We went from low-fat to low-carbohydrate, to the high protein diet. It is no wonder we end up confused with what food to eat and what to avoid. One can only imagine what the next diet craze will be and which nutrient will be outed as a villain next.

A 2017 Food and Health survey by the International Food Information Council (IFIC) reported that 78% of the respondents believe they encountered confusing information about what food to eat; 56% say the conflicting information made them doubt the choices they make. These doubts, in turn, make it difficult for people to sort all the conflicting and inconsistent information they get from different sources.

This does not mean that all sources of information about healthy foods are not trustworthy. You have to sift through all the sources and look for the most credible and evidence-based information about food. More often than not, healthy eating is not about a single excellent nutrient, but the combination of nutrients and a change in dietary pattern.

Healthy eating should give you the nutrients needed to be healthy, have energy, and feel good. This book is divided into six chapters which discuss the nutrients needed for healthy eating.

Chapter 1 covers the basic principles of changing what you eat.

This chapter presents the basic principles of a healthy diet, focusing on what food to eat. It discusses what you need for healthy eating, using the principles of a healthy diet to guide you in your choice of food. It also presents information on the essential nutrients to help you arrive at an informed decision.

Chapter 2 is about what whole, real food is, the benefits we get from eating whole food, what food to eat and what food to avoid.

The focus of healthy eating has been on individual macronutrients. We hear about carbohydrates (low-carb diet) and fats (low-fat diets), but only as individual nutrients. We don't hear about them in combination with other nutrients. Recent advances in scientific research have proven that focusing too much on one nutrient is a bad idea. Shifting towards real food is a better choice for a healthy diet.

Chapter 3 is about how to keep blood sugar low

This chapter deals with the low-glycemic diet, or the low-glycemic index diet. This diet emphasizes unprocessed foods, complex carbohydrates, and food combinations. The chapter provides a brief description of what the low-glycemic diet is, its purpose, and the glycemic (GL) values. The chapter also differentiates two types of value indicators, including the low-glycemic index diet, and the low-glycemic load diet. It ends with recommendations on what low-glycemic foods you should eat and what foods to avoid.

Chapter 4 is about a scientific approach to eating healthy fats

This chapter focuses on fats, premised on the fact that not all fats are "bad fats" like we were told. In this chapter, you'll also learn about the different fats and why healthy fats are important to us. The chapter ends with recommendations for healthy fat foods you can eat and what to avoid.

Chapter 5 is about the role of protein in your health

This chapter gives a brief description of protein. Much of what we understand about protein is due to our focus on individual nutrients, forgetting that the effectiveness of protein comes from the protein package. When you consume protein, you take in other nutrients too. The protein package is discussed as well. The chapter ends with recommendations on protein foods you should have in your meals and what foods to avoid.

Chapter 6 is about the urgent need for regenerative agriculture.

The mindless use of technology in agriculture has destroyed our topsoil. This chapter deals with restoring the health of soil through regenerative agriculture. It presents farming practices which should be adapted to restore the health of our topsoil. It presents the benefits we gain through regenerative agriculture, including the ability to grow organic, healthy food.

Thanks again for downloading this book. I hope you enjoy it!

Chapter 1

Basic Principles of Changing What You Eat

Social media has made it easy for anyone to pass on information about almost anything, including nutrition science. With the growing interest in healthy food, different food products, and food diet programs, much information about food that floats around the web all claims to be clean and healthy. Each food product and food diet regimen comes in attractive advertising packages so that one cannot help but try the product or enter the diet program. We have this mindset that when the product or diet program fails to meet expectations, there are always others to choose from. In the process of changing what we eat, we fail to see that food is food and that the fault may not be in the food per se, but in our dietary pattern. Further, despite the appearance of a wide variety of food products and food diet programs, the basic principles of healthy eating remain the same. Principles of a healthy diet

Adequacy

The food you eat should be adequate to provide the body with the nutrients needed for energy, the body's optimal growth, the ability to maintain cells, organs, and tissue. These nutrients are water, fats, carbohydrates, proteins, vitamins, and minerals. When you move about to perform your daily tasks and activities, the nutrients you have taken in through your diet get spent and you need to replenish them with the food you eat. Furthermore, you need the proper amount of these nutrients to avoid deficiencies.

Calorie Control

Knowing what to eat is not enough to make up healthy eating. You need to know how much – nutrition-wise - you are eating. You might eat healthy food, but overindulging would defeat the purpose of eating healthy. Eat food with a reasonable allowance for calorie intake. The amount of energy the body receives through food intake should be matched with how much energy the body needs to sustain its physiological and biological activities. If the energy received and spent is not balanced, it can lead to weight gain or weight loss.

Nutritional Density

Another principle in healthy eating is to eat food that contains the most nutrients with the least amount of calories. For instance, beef liver and steak contain a large number of nutrients. Between the two, however, the liver has more nutrients and has fewer calories. Since beef liver has more nutrients and fewer calories, it is more nutrient-dense. Monitoring calorie intake by the number will not be useful enough. An example is where you have a can of soda and a bowl of grapes. Both may have the same number of calories. The grapes, however, contain more nutrients than the cola and should be the fitting choice, especially if you are trying to lose weight.

Balance

Having a balanced diet means eating food which contains sufficient nutrients from each class of food. For instance, milk is a great source of calcium and protein and iron can come from fish. However, they are not sufficient for a balanced diet. You need other nutrients to balance your diet, like carbohydrates, fats, and vitamins obtained from other food sources. To achieve a balanced diet is to have a sufficient amount of servings from a variety of types of food.

Variety

There are individuals who can eat the same food for a length of time. Having a variety of food, however, is what makes eating interesting and inviting. It is possible to eat many different foods as long as the nutrients the foods contain are balanced and nutrient-dense.

Moderation

Some health and weight-conscious individuals follow diet programs with too many restrictions on what food they can and cannot eat. Following food restrictions often makes it difficult for these individuals to pursue sensible eating. We have been led to believe for so long that fatty foods are bad for our health. This belief, though misguided, influenced consumers to stay away from fats. However, not all fatty foods are bad.

The essentials of a healthy diet

There has been a growing concern with calorie intake, and people are obsessed with reducing their calories to maintain weight and improve health. Monitoring the number of calories you consume has its merits, but it is not enough to sustain the body and repair tissues damaged during activities.

What makes for healthy eating is a healthy dietary regimen that puts emphasis on whole grain foods, vegetables, and fruits. Further, you should also limit the intake of refined starches, dairy products, and beverages high in sugars.

Maintaining a healthy dietary pattern has the benefit of reducing the risk of various chronic diseases. Below are evidence-based elements of nutrition that are healthy.

Healthy Fat

The belief that fats lead to a variety of chronic diseases made fatty foods a very misunderstood and maligned nutrient. This myth has been with us for so long -- since the 1960s – and many marketers and developers of diet programs have capitalized on the misinformation. The myth, however, is an oversimplification of an important nutrient. The fact that fat-free foods are rich in calories and carbohydrates is being ignored. The oversimplification of fat-free food diets led to two negative health consequences: obesity and type 2 diabetes.

There is no evidence to suggest that dietary fat is linked to chronic diseases. Fats are healthy for you if you reduce your consumption of harmful fats and focus on healthy fats.

Carbohydrates

It was mentioned already that the fear of fatty foods led to the increase in carbohydrate intake, which most often, came from consuming processed grains. Processing food removes fiber, minerals, healthy fats, vitamins, and other nutrients. Food processing, therefore, has the effect of making us nutrient-deficient.

Too much intake of processed food leads to the increase of triglycerides and the decrease in HDL. These effects are adverse to one's health, especially regarding sensitivity to insulin and the susceptibility to type 2 diabetes.

Glycemic Index

Glycemic index refers to the increase in blood sugar because of a persons carbohydrate intake. When you take in carbohydrates through the food you consume, sugar is typically also consumed. The higher the post-meal spike in sugar, the higher the food's glycemic index. A food with a high glycemic index is refined grain, for example.

Consuming refined grains leads to a rapid and much higher overall increase in blood sugar than less-refined whole grains. A high glycemic response, which often appears with a heightened level of plasma insulin, is believed to be one cause of metabolic syndrome and ovulatory infertility.

Refined grains are processed grains. When a grain is processed, it loses the fiber and micronutrients the body needs. It is this loss which contributes to the adverse health effects.

Unprocessed whole grains, foods sourced from whole grains, together with fruits and vegetables are slow to digest by contrast. They make you feel full longer. They are also rich in fiber, vitamins, phytonutrients, and minerals which reduce the risk of cardiovascular disease and other adverse health effects.

Protein

New evidence in nutrition science shows that there are two sides to carbohydrates and fats. The same is true with protein; there is more to this nutrient than we know. Further, it does not matter whether we get our protein from plant or animal sources.

What is important to know is that protein comes in a package comprising carbohydrates, fats, minerals, vitamins and other nutrients. And, the contents of the protein package are what contributes to long-term health.

Vegetables and Fruits

"Eat your fruits and vegetables." It has been drilled into us since childhood. We always hear they are healthy for us. Vegetables and fruits have a place in one's diet due to their concentration of minerals, vitamins, phytochemicals, and fiber. Daily meals should include an abundance of fruits and vegetables which help protect against cardiovascular diseases, macular degeneration, impaired vision due to cataracts, and maintain bowel function.

Beverages

Water should be able to provide 100% of the body's needs. The other beverages which are safe to consume are coffee and tea. Beverages which become problematic are those rich in sugar (fruit drinks, sodas, and sports drinks to mention a few) and alcohol. Drinking too many sweetened beverages is linked to obesity, type 2 diabetes, gout, and heart disease. Sometimes, consumption of sweetened beverages and alcohol can lead to cancer.

Vitamins and Minerals

Vitamins and minerals are contained in the healthy food we eat. However, most people do not follow an optimal diet. Supplements are, therefore, taken to compensate for the lack of naturally sourced vitamins and minerals.

Conclusion

The basic principles of eating a healthy diet from a scientific standpoint are straightforward. It starts with making sure you are receiving an adequate amount of essential nutrients the body needs to be healthy. Next is making sure you don't get too much of a good thing. Calorie control is important for a healthy diet. Nutritional density is the next basic principle. Eating foods that are highly nutritious rather than nutritionally void helps our bodies get all the nutrients they need. There is a balancing act constantly going on in our bodies in innumerable ways. Eating a balanced diet helps our bodies stay healthy by not having to overcompensate for our out of balance diet. Variety is a key principle to a healthy diet. Eating weird foods that we don't normally come across supplies us with nutrients and combinations of nutrients that we don't find other places. Finally, moderation keeps us from eating too much of one food and eating too little of another.

The essential things that you need to pay attention to for a healthy diet are healthy fats, carbohydrates, the glycemic index of the foods you eat, protein, fruits and vegetables, the beverages you drink, and the vitamins and minerals you are getting from foods or multivitamins. Paying attention to your intake of these essentials will keep you healthy and we will look at them from a scientific standpoint in the following chapters.

Foods you should avoid

- Foods with additives
- Meats with antibiotics

- Meats with hormones
- Fruits and vegetables with pesticides
- GMO fruits and vegetables
- Processed foods
- Foods that come in packages like cans and plastics with
- BPA and Phthalates

Chapter 2

More Than the Sum of Individual Nutrients

The focus on individual nutrients contributing to health began as early as the 1930s. It was when Vitamin C was identified as being contained in citrus fruits. Vitamin C is beneficial in preventing scurvy. Research on the significance of individual nutrients to health continued. However, new evidence has surfaced reinforcing the notion that healthy food is more than the sum of individual nutrients. Food research conducted has proven that the focus on the individual nutrient was misguided. A much better approach to healthy eating is food synergy, which claims health benefits are provided, not by a single nutrient, but by a combination of compounds that work more effectively together than as separates.

Because of these food studies, we are seeing a shift to whole food.

What are whole real foods?

Stated simply, real food is food in its original and natural form and has not been altered. Real food has not been processed and contains no additives.

Real food is the food our early ancestors ate as part of their diet. This dietary pattern changed with the introduction of ready-to-eat food which became popular in the 21st century. Ready-to-eat food may be convenient for people in a rush, but they lack the compounds that contribute to a healthier and happier life.

What do we get from whole food?

Phytochemicals – This is a class of compounds which contain powerful antioxidants, like lycopene found in tomatoes, anthocyanins sourced from berries, and pterostilbene which breaks down fats and cholesterol in cells. You have consumed phytochemicals if you consume unprocessed plant vegetables and fruit.

Loads of Nutrients– Health surveys show that people today get too little vitamin C, D, and A, and the minerals potassium, and magnesium. Deficiency in nutrients can develop into chronic diseases like heart disease, cancer, diabetes, and high blood pressure. Nutrient deficiencies are addressed by eating whole foods rich in nutrients.

Good fats – Fats have long earned a bad name through misinformation. There are, however, good fats which our body's need as a major source of energy. By eating whole food, you eliminate the bad fats which you find in abundance in fast foods and processed foods. Good fats are sourced from whole foods, like vegetables, fish, and fruits. One important good fat is Omega 3 which is obtained from fish and plants.

Fiber – When you eat whole plant foods with enough variety, you won't need supplements. Whole foods provide the body with the needed fiber to keep blood glucose down, help the body feel full longer since fiber digests slowly, and lowers the risk of heart disease and diabetes.

Fewer additives in food – Whole foods are natural foods without the additives found in processed foods, like sodium and sugar, and artificial color.

Whole grains – Whole grains, unlike the common belief, offer more than just fiber. When you eat whole grains, you get a package of nutrients which provide many more benefits health-wise. For instance, whole grain reduces the risk for diabetes by lowering blood glucose and sensitivity to insulin.

Whole real foods you can eat

- Vegetables and fruits (preferably organic)
- Organic dairy
- Whole grains
- Fish free of chemicals
- Meat sourced from organic or grass-fed animals
- Unrefined sweeteners, such as maple syrup and honey
- Poultry, legumes, seeds, nut that are, again, organic

Foods to avoid

Avoid eating processed foods with no nutritional value. Processed foods are the ready-to-eat foods high in calories, fat, and sugar. Examples of foods to avoid are:

- Snack foods with high calories, like cheese snacks and chips
- Convenience foods, such as pizza and frozen dinners
- Boxed meal mixes which are rich in sodium and bad fats
- White rice, white pasta, and white bread

- Canned foods loaded with sodium
- Breakfast cereals rich in sugar
- Soft drinks

Chapter 3

Keep Blood Sugar Low

Sugar is an addictive substance. So much so that studies have shown that Oreo's are more addictive to rats than cocaine is in tests. The average person consumes about 152 pounds (69 kg) of sugar every year. It is the number one contributor to obesity, type II diabetes, heart disease, dementia, and cancer. High fructose corn syrup contributes to 15% of the average person's calorie intake every year. Sugar-sweetened beverages are the number one contributor to obesity. Carbohydrates are not the enemy of a healthy diet, but they have to be kept in balance, like the other macro-nutrients.

Many popular diet plans offer a regimen claiming to be effective for weight loss or maintaining health. Of these diets, research shows that some are better than others for the metabolic rate of the body.

There are three popular diet plans today: the low-carb diet, low-fat diet, and the low-glycemic (GI) diet. Of the three diet plans found to be effective, as far as metabolism is concerned, the low-glycemic diet is the best at maintaining health.

What is low glycemic diet?

A low-glycemic diet is a diet plan that helps maintain health by reducing the blood sugar and insulin levels. It shows how the food you eat affects your blood sugar levels. The GI diet is also known as a low-glycemic index diet which refers to a diet plan that uses the index as the primary guide for planning a meal.

The purpose of the glycemic index diet is to consume food containing carbohydrates that do not cause an increase in your blood sugar. This diet plan monitors the number of carbohydrates consumed by assigning a GI value to carbohydrates.

The GI values are divided into 3 categories:

Low GI –1 to 55

Medium GI – 56 to 69

High GI – 70 and up

Using the GI values gives you an idea about your choice of healthy food. For instance, a muffin made of white wheat flour has a GI value of 77 while a whole wheat muffin has a GI value of 45. The lower the GI value, the healthier the food consumed. A low-glycemic index, however, has its limitations because it does not take into consideration the number of carbohydrates in a particular food.

Another way to determine low-glycemic diet is the low-glycemic load.

Low-glycemic load ranks food rich in carbohydrates by measuring how many carbohydrates are contained in a food serving. A low-glycemic load is considered a better predictor of eating healthy food than the low-glycemic index. A low-glycemic load score has the following range:

Low GL – 10 or less

Medium GL – 11 to 19

High GL – 20 up

Low-glycemic foods you can eat:

Non-starchy vegetables – most vegetables have low GL levels from 1 to 7. You can include lettuce, spinach, broccoli, artichokes, onion, green beans, peppers, and other leafy greens in your meals.

Nuts and seeds – these food types have low GL ranging from 1 to 17 per serving, with cashew nuts having the highest score. You can include chia seeds, pumpkin seeds, walnuts, flaxseeds, and almonds in your meals.

Whole grains - The GL score for whole grains ranges from 10 to 17. Choose whole grains that are minimally processed. You can eat brown rice, steel-cut oats, sprouted grain bread, muesli, granola, and whole wheat pasta.

Beans and legumes – The GL scores for these vegetables range from 2 to 13 per serving. Soybeans and chickpeas are good choices.

Yogurt and other fermented dairy – Dairy products have a GL score ranging from 1 to 5. Try yogurt that is plain and unsweetened. You can also have the raw whole milk.

Fresh fruit – GL score for fruits range between 4 and 14. You can eat cherries, apples, berries, citrus fruits. It is okay to have up to 3 servings of fresh fruits in your meals daily. Choose fresh fruits instead of fruit juice.

Healthy fats – Pure fats and oils have no carbohydrates and, therefore, contain zero GL score. Use extra virgin olive oil, virgin coconut oil, and MCT oil.

Quality proteins - Animal proteins have zero GL score. You can eat free-range eggs, salmon fish, grass-fed lamb or beef, pasture-raised poultry, and raw dairy products.

Carbohydrates and Grains

You cannot talk about keeping blood sugar low without also addressing carbohydrates from the grains we eat today. It is only within the last 200 years we have eaten the refined grains we see today. Now we are eating an average of 133 pounds of flour per person every year. It has only been during the last 10,000 years of human history that grains have had any significant role in our diet. That may sound like a long time, but not long enough for us to adapt to the effects that grain has on our bodies.
In that 10,000 years, we have changed the grain we eat as well. Through the agricultural manipulation of crossbreeding of grains with other grains and grasses, we have ended up with dwarf hybridized wheat. This wheat is not like the wheat of 10,000 years ago and is far worse for our health. It contains inflammatory proteins and proteins that are addictive. The processed flour we eat today actually has a glycemic index higher than that of table sugar. It's hard to believe, but eating bread will affect your

blood glucose more than eating table sugar.

Carbohydrates and Fruits and Vegetables

One area that people have trouble with when reducing their carbohydrate intake is with fruits and vegetables. Fruits and vegetables are beneficial in the right quantities of the right kind, but they can be counterproductive if you are eating low-glycemic foods. The top 5 vegetables that Americans eat are potatoes (in the form of french fries), tomatoes (in the form of ketchup and pizza sauce), sweet corn (which is full of starch), onions, and iceberg lettuce. You can see that this list of vegetables is neither very nutritionally dense nor very low-glycemic.

When you consume the right fruits and vegetables, on the other hand, you receive phytochemicals that have the power to fight disease, regulate the microbiome in your gut, work as antioxidants and anti-inflammatory agents, and detoxify your body. It is important to pick fruit and vegetables that contain high levels of vitamins, minerals, and fiber. You should also pick fruits and vegetables that are in a wide range of colors. Flavonoids are compounds in fruits and vegetables which make up their color. There is a great deal of ongoing research regarding flavonoids and their anti-inflammatory, antioxidant, cancer reducing, and cardiovascular health properties. The best way to get all the benefits from flavonoids is to "eat the rainbow" of fruits and vegetables.

When eating fruit, focus on berries and other low-glycemic fruits. Also focus on eating fatty fruits like avocados, olives, and coconut. These contain lots of vitamins and minerals without increasing your carbohydrate intake. Avoid fruit juice as this takes out all the beneficial fiber you would get from fruit and leaves you with all the sugar.

If you cannot buy organic fruits and vegetables it is important to know about the dirty dozen and avoid them. There are fruits and vegetables that are the worst when it comes to pesticides. They include strawberries, spinach, nectarines, apples, grapes, peaches, cherries, pears, tomatoes, celery, potatoes, and bell peppers.

Conclusion

Sugar is one of the leading causes of many of the diseases we see today. It has to be kept in check, like the other macro-nutrients, for us to have a healthy diet. Of all the diets out there, current research tells us that the low-glycemic diet is one of the best for losing weight and maintaining health. This diet does not demonize carbohydrates or sugar, it simply limits how much you take in, and focuses on foods that have the least effect on blood sugar.

There are two ways of going about a low-glycemic diet. One is the use of the glycemic index for foods, the other is to use the glycemic load for foods. Using the glycemic load is the better method of the two.
One of the main problems we see today as far as carbohydrates in our diets go is refined grains. These come from grains we have engineered and affect blood sugar more than eating sugar itself. These refined grains and flours contribute to a wide range of diseases.

Make sure you eat lots of fruits and vegetables, but not the typical five that Americans eat. Eat the rainbow to get the most benefits from them and focus on low-glycemic fruits and vegetables.

Healthy glycemic foods you can eat:

- Whole grains, milled whole grains
- Gluten-free grains like black rice, and red rice
- Quinoa, wild rice, amaranth, buckwheat, etc.
- Rye, barley, and other gluten-containing grains sparingly
- Low-glycemic, organic fruits, and vegetables

Foods you should avoid for a low-glycemic index diet:

- Refined grains and flour, which includes packaged grain products, white wheat flour, packaged cereal products, and other foods sourced from refined grains and flour.
- Sweetened beverages, such as bottled juices and sodas.
- Table sugar, molasses, etc.
- Dried fruits, such as dates and raisins.
- Starchy root vegetables, like white potatoes in limited quantities.
- Gluten-free foods containing sugar and refined grains
- The dirty dozen fruits and vegetables

Chapter 4

A Scientific Approach to Eating Healthy Fats

Just the mention of fats produces a negative response from most people, believing all fats are harmful to our health. Recent research, however, shows that fats are as harmful as we once thought.

Fats are molecules comprising carbon and hydrogen elements which are joined by long chains known as hydrocarbons. It is how the molecular structure of fats form that determines whether the fats are healthy or not healthy. Healthy fats are those foods that are relatively unprocessed and sourced from whole foods. Monounsaturated and polyunsaturated fats are healthy fats.

Types of fats

Trans fats – these type of fats come from hydrogenated oils and are bad for the cardiovascular system, as well as the other parts of the body. These fats are man-made and increase harmful low-density lipoprotein (LDL) cholesterol. Not only do trans fats increase LDL, but they can destroy high-density lipoprotein (HDL) cholesterol which protects the body from harmful health effects, like damage to arteries.

Further, high intake of trans fats is found to lead to several risk factors, such as the cardiovascular disease, gallstones, type 2 diabetes, weight gain, and dementia.

Saturated fats –These fats are sourced from red

meats and dairy products. New research findings show that a combination of different foods which contain nutrients, fatty acids, and bioactives modifies the effects of saturated fats on corollary heart disease (CHD). Instead of focusing on the amount of saturated fat consumed, the focus should be on the food source, grass-fed for example.

Monounsaturated and polyunsaturated fats – Both of these fats are found in vegetable oils, seeds, nuts, fish, and whole grains. Considered to be the most important of these fats is the polyunsaturated omega-3 fatty acid found to be significant for cardiac health. The effect of eating polyunsaturated fats, in place of saturated fats and trans fats, significantly increases the chances of improving sensitivity to insulin. Polyunsaturated fats also have the capacity to stabilize irregular heart rhythms.

The importance of healthy fats

Our body needs fats. The fats we get from the food we consume gives our body energy which enables us to work and keep our hair and skin healthy. Fats also help our body absorb vitamins A, D, E, and K since they are not water soluble.

Fats provide our system with the essential fatty acids known as linoleic (omega 6) and linolenic (omega 3) acids necessary for our metabolism, maintenance of health, body tissues, hormone production, cell signaling, enhancement of our immune system, and the absorption of the nutrients the body needs.

Among the health benefits we get from consuming fats are:

- Protection from the risk of cardiovascular diseases

- Improved body composition
- Easing of depression
- Prevention of cancer
- Preservation of eye health
- Reduction in aggressive behavior
- Reduction of ADD and ADHD symptoms

The misconception about fat

You are what you eat as the saying goes. If we eat a diet rich in fatty foods then, likewise, we will be rich in fat. At least that is what we were told. Low-fat diets have been all the rage for decades. These diets were not backed by science though. What science tells us is quite the opposite. When we include more healthy fats in our diet, our bodies get healthier.

One scientific review published in The Lancet Diabetes & Endocrinology in 2015 looked at 53 randomized controlled trials on diet and weight loss that lasted a year or more. The review found that higher fat diets outperformed low-fat diets. It also found that low-fat diets only had more weight loss than the normal American diet when compared to the other diets in the 53 trials. So we aren't what we eat after all and a diet rich in fat promotes weight loss rather than weight gain.

Another scientific review published in PLOS One in 2016 looked at butter consumption and health. This review looked at 9 different studies which included 636,000 people. This review found that there was no link between butter consumption and heart disease. In fact, it found a link between butter consumption and a lower risk of having type II diabetes.

Another interesting study was done in 2016 on recovered data from an experiment which occurred between 1968 and 1973. This was published in The BMJ and looked at data collected regarding vegetable oil consumption and health. The original experiment used over 9,000 participants. The study found that people consuming vegetable oil had a drop in their LDL cholesterol (the bad cholesterol) levels. But despite lowering their LDLs, they were found to have the highest risk of heart attack and death. In fact, for every 30mg/dl LDLs dropped in the blood, the risk of heart attack increased by 22%.

Conclusion

It turns out that fat is not so bad for us, but in fact is great for us if it comes from the right foods. There is a variety of health benefits that come from eating healthy fats, which can include, protection from the risk of cardiovascular diseases, improved body composition, easing of depression, prevention of cancer, preservation of eye health, a reduction of the incidence of aggressive behavior, a reduction of ADD and ADHD symptoms. High-fat diets help people lose weight. Butter has no link to heart disease and reduces the risk of having type II diabetes. Fats from the wrong sources (vegetable oils, and hydrogenated oils) can be very harmful to our health.

Healthy fat foods you can eat

You are safe with fats if you source them from unprocessed, whole, and high-quality foods. These healthy foods should include:

- Plant-based whole food fat
- Avocados
- Nuts: Brazil nuts, walnuts, pecans, cashews,

almonds, hazelnuts, macadamia nuts
- Seeds: hemp, chia, pumpkin, sesame, flax
- Coconut oil, extra virgin olive oil, avocado oil, MCT oil
- Pasture-raised eggs
- Wild small fish or S.M.A.S.H. fish (explained later)
- Grass-fed meats
- Pasture-raised eggs
- Grass-fed butter and ghee
- Lard, tallow, and duck fat

Fats you should avoid
- Stay away from fatty processed foods
- Factory farmed meats are likely to contain high levels of omega 6s
- Artificially created fats like hydrogenated oils
- Refined bean and seed oils containing trans fats
- Limit peanuts

Chapter 5

Protein and Your Health

We have protein in all of our systems and tissues. There are countless proteins in our bodies that make us what we are and keep us that way.

Including protein-rich food in the diet has no ideal amount or an optimal health target for calories in protein consumption. However, health and nutrition experts recommend 0.36 grams of protein per pound (0.8 grams of protein per kilogram) of body weight per day.

What is protein?

Protein is created by our bodies from building blocks known as amino acids which are made either from scratch or through modification. The essential amino acids, however, have to be sourced from foods we eat.

We typically get our essential amino acids from animal sources. Other sources, like vegetables, fruits, nuts, seeds, and grains may not have the complete essential amino acid profile our body needs.

If you are a vegetarian, you need to note this, as you may lack the essential amino acids necessary to sustain your body. There are nine amino acids (the essential amino acids) that the body cannot make on its own. It is possible to get them all from plants, but it takes planning. For example, a serving of beans and rice contains all nine essential amino acids. No wonder so many cultures have paired these two plant foods together.

The misconception about red meat

As mentioned earlier, focusing on a single nutrient is a misguided belief. New research evidence shows that a combination of elements is more effective in sustaining our health and in protecting us from the risk of chronic diseases. The same characteristic is found with protein. What makes protein sources more effective are the other nutrients they contain. Healthy or unhealthy fats, whether the package contains beneficial fiber, vitamins, minerals, and other nutrients determine the protein package. To give you an idea of the effect of the protein package – a steak from a cow that was grain fed on a CAFO (concentrated animal feeding operation) has a much lower omega 3 fatty acid content than compared to a steak from a grass-fed cow.

The body requires both omega 6s and omega 3s to function, but there is a balancing act that needs to occur between the two to remain healthy. The current recommendation for omega 6s to omega 3s is 4:1 or less. Anti-aging experts believe the ratio should be no more than 1:1. In either case, a study published in The American Journal of Clinical Nutrition in 2000 found that people consume a ratio of omega 6s to omega 3s anywhere between 12:1 and 25:1. This is why choosing the right source for your protein matters so much.

One of the major misconceptions about protein is about the saturated fat that often accompanies it in red meat. We have been told for as long as we can remember that saturated fats are the enemy and that you will have a heart attack if you eat too many of these artery-clogging fats. It turns out that this is completely false.

A study published in Food and Nutrition Research in 2016 has debunked this idea. The study covered 42 European countries, tracked 62 food items of participants and the information gathered spanned from 1993 to 2008. It was not a small study. In this study, the researchers found that the highest correlation between any food and cardiovascular disease (CVD) was in foods containing high amounts of carbohydrates and cereal grains. Contrary to popular wisdom, the researchers also found that the foods with the lowest correlation to cardiovascular disease were animal fat and animal protein. The study concluded by saying:

> "Our results do not support the association between CVDs and saturated fat, which is still contained in official dietary guidelines. Instead, they agree with data accumulated from recent studies that link CVD risk with the high glycemic index/load of carbohydrate-based diets. In the absence of any scientific evidence connecting saturated fat with CVDs, these findings show that current dietary recommendations regarding CVDs should be seriously reconsidered."

The misconception about eggs

Eggs are another source of protein that has gotten a bad wrap. The 2015 dietary guidelines state that cholesterol is no longer a nutrient of concern. All this time we thought cholesterol would give us a heart attack too. Despite the change in the dietary guidelines, many people still believe cholesterol is bad, and therefore, so are eggs. Apparently, most of us don't get the yearly memo on dietary guideline changes.

The tragedy here is that eggs are one of the true super foods out there. Not like the superfoods we see in the stores with the big colorful labels to tell us they are superfoods. Eggs aren't exotic, they aren't new and they are a cheap source of protein. They don't exactly fit into the superfood marketing scheme.

What makes an egg a superfood is all the nutrients you get out of one small package. One large egg contains 9% RDA (recommended daily allowance) of vitamin B12, 15% RDA of vitamin B2, 6% RDA of vitamin A, 7% RDA of vitamin B5, and 22% RDA of selenium. In addition, an egg also contains small amounts of nearly every vitamin and mineral essential for good health. These include calcium, iron, potassium, zinc, manganese, vitamin E, folate and many others. An egg also contains 115 mg (21% RDA) of choline, an important nutrient needed for cognitive function.

The egg is also one of the most perfect sources of protein. It's not only important to get all the essential amino acids, but it is also important to get them in the right ratios as well. Eggs have the perfect ratio of amino acids for our bodies to use them with maximum efficiency. The biological value of a food measures protein quality. Eggs have a perfect score of 100 for biological value and other foods are often measured against eggs for their biological values.

Eggs contain two powerful antioxidants called lutein and zeaxanthin. These antioxidants are known for protecting the eyes against damage from sunlight. They also reduce the risk of macular degeneration and cataracts, which are leading causes of sight impairment and blindness in elderly people.

The misconception about fish

Is fish a healthy food to eat or not? We know that some fish contain high levels of mercury. Some are being over-fished. Some are farm raised, but fed grains full of antibiotics and chemicals. There are stories of people getting parasites from eating sushi. Spawning grounds for fish like salmon have been dammed up, reducing populations. Yet we also know fish is high in omega 3s and several other important nutrients for good health. Fish seem to be one of the most confusing foods to eat in a healthy, environmentally responsible diet.

Choosing the right fish can be difficult, but when done correctly, fish are a great source of nutrients for a healthy body. Fish are a great way to increase omega 3 fatty acids which, as we looked at earlier, we need a lot more of. They also contain significant quantities of iodine, selenium, vitamin D and vitamin B12. Fish are a great source of clean protein as well.

The trick to getting all these great nutrients without the things that negatively affect your health (like mercury) is to pick the right fish. The first, and easiest way to select fish is to buy S.M.A.S.H. fish. These are wild caught salmon, mackerel, anchovies, sardines, herring. Each of these fish is fatty and high in omega 3s. Since they are also on the smaller side, they don't run the risk of containing high levels of mercury like swordfish. Shellfish like shrimp, scallops, oysters, and mussels are also great choices.

A great resource for finding fish sustainably sourced and health-wise is from the Monterey Bay Aquarium. Their site,

http://www.seafoodwatch.org/seafood-recommendations/consumer-guides

contains brochures for various regions and what fish are the best choices to choose, what fish are good alternatives, and what fish you should avoid in that particular area.

Conclusion

Protein is one of the macro-nutrients essential for our bodies to function. It can come from a myriad of sources, but the easiest and most effective source is from animals. There have been a lot of misconceptions about meat which have confused people about what is healthy to eat and what is not. It turns out that the saturated fat in red meat and the cholesterol in eggs are not linked to cardiovascular disease after all. It is important to choose protein sources that have been pasture-raised and grass fed, however because of the omega 3 content in them. Eggs are a true superfood containing almost every nutrient we need to survive in some quantity. Finally, fish a great source of protein, but they are confusing. If we stick to S.M.A.S.H. fish or use the guides provided by the Monterey Bay Aquarium, however, it is much easier to find healthy fish to eat.

Protein food sources you can eat:

- Pasture-raised poultry (duck, turkey, chicken)
- Grass-fed dairy products like yogurt, and milk as a

treat
- Cheese
- Eggs from pasture-raised hens
- Low glycemic beans (smaller beans like lentils, navy, etc.)
- Red meats that have been grass fed
- S.M.A.S.H. fish (wild salmon, mackerel, anchovies, sardines, herring)
- Shellfish including shrimp, scallops, oysters, and mussels

Foods to avoid

- Meats from concentrated animal feeding operations (CAFOs)
- Antibiotic and hormone-treated meats
- Tuna, swordfish, Chilean sea bass, halibut, grouper
- Farmed fish that is not organic or sustainably raised
- CAFO dairy products
- Kidney, lima, and fava beans

Chapter 6

The Urgent Need for Regenerative Agriculture

The trend in healthy eating is going back to what is natural and organic with food. But, do we know what is behind the concept of organic food?

Driving down a country road in some places, you will see miles of soy fields or corn crops. The abundance of food crops can amaze you. However, what you see is the use of the monoculture system of farming which is detrimental to the soil, and heavily impacts nature and biodiversity in the area.

A better approach is regenerative agriculture.

Why Regenerative Agriculture?

Throughout history, man has depended on the earth's resources for survival. Of these resources, man, through agriculture, made use of soil and water to produce food for sustenance. Soil and water are indispensable for our plant and animal-based food production system. Indeed, agriculture has supported human society in all of its cycle of development.

We cannot deny the critical role of agriculture in human society, but its use has disrupted the natural ecosystems. Modern agriculture has adversely affected our soil systems, water systems, animal populations, and plant communities.

Soil degradation is a natural process, but this has been intensified by pollution and pollutants caused by human activity. In agriculture, soil degradation occurs due to:

Improper cultivation practices. Several of the agricultural practices widely used today are detrimental to the environment and considered to be the biggest contributor to the decline of the soil quality. One main factor for soil degradation is tillage which breaks the soil into particles, increasing erosion rate. The mechanization of agriculture aggravated the decline of soil quality due to deep plowing, and the loss of plant cover. Other cultivation practices that damage the soil are steep slope farming, mono-cropping, surface irrigation, and row-cropping.

Overgrazing. This is another farming practice which contributes to soil degradation. Overgrazing has the same destructive effects to the soil as the improper cultivation.

Excess use or misuse of fertilizers. The misuse and excessive use of chemical fertilizers and pesticides kill the organisms that facilitate binding of the soil. Further, the improper use of pesticides and fertilizers kills the soils micro-organisms and beneficial bacteria that contribute to soil formation.

Deforestation. Deforestation leads to soil degradation due to the exposure of soil minerals when trees and crop cover are removed. Trees support the litter layers and humus on the soil's surface necessary for soil formation and for binding the soil together.

Soil degradation results in:

- Land degradation
- Aridity and drought
- Loss of arable land
- Flooding
- Pollution and clogged waterways

What is regenerative Agriculture?

Regenerative agriculture is the opposite of the monoculture system. It is a blanket term that refers to farming and grazing practices that help reverse climate change through rebuilding organic matter and restoring soil biodiversity. Besides the carbon draw-down, this practice also helps to improve the water cycle.

The mechanization of agriculture has destroyed our topsoil due to poor soil management, erosion, and intensive chemical use. With the rate we are degrading our soil, we can expect the topsoil to be gone in 60 years according to Maria-Helena Semedo of the Food and Agriculture Organization (FAO), a specialized branch of the United Nations. With our topsoil gone, so will our agriculture be. It used to be that sustainable agriculture was the buzzword. But, this was empty of meaning. The term "regenerative" was used instead, which was more indicative of its purpose in agriculture. What is more important is that the choice of the word "regenerative" puts emphasis on building soil health.

Building soil health is accomplished through the following farming and grazing practices:

- No tilling/minimum tilling.

- Restoration of soil fertility through crop rotation, cover crops, animal manures, and compost
- Use of full-time inter-crop planting, multiple crop planting, multi-species cover crops, bee and other beneficial insect habitat built on planted borders.
- Well-managed grazing practices

The benefits we get from regenerative agriculture if we, as a global community, recognize the urgent need to preserve our soil, we can:

- Feed the world
- Reduce GHG emissions. Today's industrial food system accounts for 44 to 57 percent of global greenhouse gas emissions. With a new food system, GHG emissions can be significantly reduced.
- Reverse climate change
- Improve agricultural yields
- Create soil that is drought-resistant
- Revitalize local economies
- Preserve agriculture's traditional knowledge
- Restore biodiversity
- Restore grasslands
- Improve nutrition

Conclusion

So much information about healthy and unhealthy food coming from those who offer different diet regimen, nutrition and health experts, and from the food marketing industry only result in confusion. As a result, consumers question the food they eat, whether the food contains healthy compounds or are harmful to their health.

New research now debunks previous eating beliefs and patterns. It is my hope that the information in this book will give you a new perspective on healthy food and a scientific approach to choosing what food to eat. A scientific approach is the way to go in living a healthy life rather than basing your decisions on what has been drilled into you since childhood. Your health might even suffer if you follow the trend and eat the food that is popular, even without understanding the basis for the choice of food.

There is a need to set aside the obsession of a single nutrient and shift attention to the combination of nutrients that accounts for the maintenance of a healthy and high performing body, which leads to a more healthy and productive life.

Be mindful of new diets as they emerge. You have to ask yourself how much science shows a diet to be successful. It is not always easy. Most diets don't show you a long list of studies proving they are healthy. You just see a lot of before and after pictures of people who have lost a lot of weight. This doesn't prove anything, only that they found people willing to get paid to be in a commercial or on their website.

I encourage you to read about diets you may want to try in the future and look for the scientific evidence to support, or debunk them. I have written books on weight loss diets and they all contain studies proving they are a healthy choice for losing weight. Avoid articles and books that only give you the success stories and guides. They are not looking out for your health. Read material citing scientific studies and you will be doing the best thing you can for your health and your body.

The next step is to change the food you eat based on the information you gained from reading this book. It will amaze you to see the changes in yourself if you start now and begin to enjoy a healthier life.

Thank you again for downloading this book!

I hope this book helps you and gives you some good information about what foods to eat to arrive at an informed, healthy choice.

Thank you and good luck!

Preview of Ketogenic Diet: Beginners Guide and
    Cookbook for Weight Loss With the Keto Diet
    & The Secret To Success That No One is
    Talking About – Ten Day Meal Plan and Fifty
    Delicious Recipes

Myths about ketogenic dieting

Now that you have seen just a few of the good
things the ketogenic diet can do for you, beyond just
helping you lose the extra weight, let's look at some of the
myths about the ketogenic diet that may be holding you
back. Once we bust these myths there shouldn't be any
reason you wouldn't want to start the ketogenic diet today.

The brain needs a constant supply of sugar

I struggled to get over this myth. The brain does
indeed need a constant supply of fuel, and most of that fuel,
in the average person comes from glucose taken in from
our food, but it does not have to. Many people believe, as I
did, that you have to eat carbohydrates in order to fuel the
brain. The body has several mechanisms to fuel the brain if
we don't eat carbohydrates for a while, or even stop eating
them all together. If you think about it, it doesn't make
sense that our hunter-gatherer ancestors would require a
constant supply of carbohydrates, otherwise their brains
would shut down, making it impossible for them to find
more food with carbohydrates. The first backup for blood
sugar that our bodies have if we don't consume
carbohydrates is in our liver. Our liver stores glycogen, a
form of glucose, which can be used for hours to power the

brain. The next backup the body has for supplying the brain with power is called gluconeogenesis. This is a process where the body produces glucose from non-carbohydrate substances like lactate, glycerol, and glucogenic amino acids. Finally, if the body undergoes a long term low carbohydrate diet, long term fasting or starvation, it can generate fuel for the brain in the form of ketone bodies from dietary fats. These ketone bodies significantly reduce the brain's need for glucose. So during a ketogenic diet the combination of ketone bodies and glucose from gluconeogenesis sustain the brain's need for energy long term. The truth is that we don't need to eat carbohydrates to fuel our brains. Our bodies have adapted to compensate for long periods with no carbohydrates in our diets. Ketogenic dieting will never overcome those compensatory mechanisms.

The ketogenic diet is just a fad diet

The ketogenic diet cannot be truthfully labeled as a fad diet. Anyone who says it is a fad diet is either ignorant of the facts or is probably trying to sell you something. As we have already seen, the ketogenic diet has been recognized for almost 100 years as a treatment for epilepsy. But going back even further, we see that low carbohydrate diets are even older still. The first low carbohydrate diet was published in 1863. At that time it saw great success too.

In addition to being such an old concept for dieting, low carbohydrate diets have been proven to work in more than 22 different scientific studies just since 2003. So we are talking about a fad that has been around more than 150 years and has a proven track record of success for people. In fact, that doesn't really sound like a fad diet at all. Fad diets may come and go every year, but the ketogenic diet is not one of them. It has been around a long time and will continue to be a successful way for people to lose weight for a long time to come.

The ketogenic diet is hard to stick to

Some say that the ketogenic diet is harder than other diets to stick to because you have to remove entire food groups from your diet. This causes a person to crave the missing food groups and they ultimately end up breaking their diet as a result. All diets cut something out though, whether that is a food group or calories. The problem with the idea that ketogenic dieting is harder to stick to, however, is that you can actually eat until you are full. People who restrict calories on the other hand do not get the luxury of ever being satisfied with a meal. That is a definite recipe for breaking your diet.

A review of 19 separate studies from 2004 to 2012 found that people were actually very successful at sticking to low carbohydrate diets. On average, there was an 80% success rate with people sticking to their low carbohydrate diets in these 19 studies. Unfortunately, there is no hard data on how many people are successful at achieving their goals through dieting, but studies show that percentages of people who stick with their calorie restricted diets are anywhere between 5% and 50%. So even if the success rate of the average dieter is 50%, though that seems unlikely, ketogenic dieting helps 30% more people to follow through with their diet. It is quite possibly the most successful diet out there when it comes to ease of sticking to it.

The ketogenic diet is bad for your heart

Since the ketogenic diet is high in fat it is assumed that it is bad for heart health. People state that the high amount of dietary fat will increase cholesterol in the blood and lead to heart disease. As we have already seen from several studies, however, triglycerides go down, HDLs go up, blood pressure decreases, and LDLs become more healthy.

In addition, a study published in 2014 in the Annals of Medicine found that low carbohydrate diets like the ketogenic diet can reduce inflammation as well. So the ketogenic diet has been shown in studies to tackle all of the major risk factors for heart disease. It is not bad for your heart, but instead is actually good for heart health.

Most weight loss comes from water weight

It is true that you will lose water weight at the beginning of the ketogenic diet. This is because the glycogen that you store in your liver and muscles, as a backup if your blood sugar gets low, binds to water. In addition, as blood sugar levels drop, so do insulin levels. This drop in insulin allows the kidneys to remove more sodium from the body resulting in less water retention as well. The result of these two factors working together will almost immediately cause a significant amount of water weight to be lost. There is no good reason to argue that this is a bad thing. If you don't need that extra five to ten pounds of water weight, why carry it around everywhere?

The loss of water weight is often used as an argument against the ketogenic diet. Some say that water weight is the only thing that is lost while on the ketogenic diet. This is totally false, however. A study published in 2002 in Metabolism: Clinical and Experimental found that participants of a six-week ketogenic diet lost an average of

7.5 pounds of fat and gained an average of 2.4 pounds of muscle.

The ketogenic diet reduces the amount of healthy fruits and vegetables you eat

The argument here is that if you cut out all of your carbohydrates, then you won't be eating any fruits or vegetables. This is a fallacy though because low-carbohydrate does not mean no-carbohydrate dieting. You might be surprised at how many fruits and vegetables you can eat and stay within the guidelines for the ketogenic diet. In fact, many people find that they tend to eat more fruits and vegetables while on the ketogenic diet because your body will start to crave them. They contain many of the vitamins and minerals, like vitamin C and potassium, that your body will need as your health increases. Once you take carbohydrates out of your meals, you will be looking to replace them with something else, and fruits and vegetables will be an easy thing to replace them with.

The ketogenic diet only works because you eat fewer calories

While it is true that the ketogenic diet will cause you to lose weight due to reduced caloric intake, that is not the whole story. The calorie reduction happens automatically on the ketogenic diet, unlike other diets. You don't have to force the reduction on yourself. In fact, when the ketogenic diet is compared with low fat and calorie restricted diets, participants lose up to two or three times as much weight. This was the conclusion of a study published in 2002 in the Journal of Clinical Endocrinology and Metabolism. This not only has to do with the fact that calorie restriction is automatic, but is also due to an increase in the metabolism. A study published in 2004 in the Journal of the American College of Nutrition found that high protein diets like the ketogenic diet speed up the metabolism, increasing weight loss compared with other diets.

The ketogenic diet will ruin your physical performance

Many people believe that carbohydrates are essential for peak physical performance. The majority of top athletes eat a high carbohydrate diet so it follows that it must be the best diet to perform at your best. It is true that your physical performance will suffer in the beginning of the ketogenic diet. This is because your body is adapting to using fat for energy. However, after you give yourself a few weeks to get used to the new changes, you will find that the ketogenic diet no longer inhibits you. Several studies have confirmed that low carbohydrate diets like the ketogenic diet improve physical performance in the long term, especially endurance activities. One such study published in 2014 in the British Journal of Sports Medicine found that as long as people are given a few weeks to adapt, they perform better while on the low carbohydrate diet. Other studies, including one published in 2014 in the Journal of the International Society of Sports Medicine, have found the low carbohydrate dieting is beneficial to muscle strength and mass.

Ketosis is a damaging metabolic state

This idea is a confusion of two different metabolic terms. Ketosis is often confused with keto**acid**osis. Ketosis is when your body synthesizes ketones from fat for fuel. Ketoacidosis is a dangerous condition that is typically caused by uncontrolled type I diabetes. Ketoacidosis is when the bloodstream is flooded with ketones to the point where it turns acidic. It can be fatal if it is not treated. You will never enter a state of ketoacidosis while on the ketogenic diet. Something has to be wrong with your body for ketoacidosis to occur.

Takeaway

As you can see from this list of myths about the ketogenic diet, there is a lot of misinformation out there. It comes from marketing ploys, fear, and ignorance. Hopefully, this list has taught you that these myths are inaccurate and rid you of any fears that you may have about starting the ketogenic diet. There is nothing to lose by trying it but the weight. The benefits of ketogenic dieting are numerous and worth the effort of trying it out.

Get the rest of *Ketogenic Diet: Beginners Guide and Cookbook for Weight Loss With the Keto Diet & The Secret To Success That No One is Talking About – Ten Day Meal Plan and Fifty Delicious Recipes* today on Amazon.

Made in the USA
San Bernardino, CA
23 June 2019